ALTERNATIVE WAYS TO MANAGE DIABETES

Merle Wilson

DEDICATION

To my son, Adrian

CONTENTS

1   INTRODUCTION   1

2   WHAT IS DIABETES   2

3   TRADITIONAL MEDICATIONS   4

4   FOCUS ON FOOD   5

5   DIETARY SUPPLEMENTS   13

6   MINERAL AND VITAMIN SUPPLEMENTS   18

7   HERBAL REMEDIES   23

8   LET'S GET PHYSICAL   27

9   SKIN   CARE   32

10   FOOT CARE   34

11   PYSHICAL TREATMENT   36

12   HOLISTIC APPROACHES   50

ACKNOWLEDGMENTS

To my family for their support in writing this book.

1 INTRODUCTION

How the body works

Our bodies require energy simply so that the major organs can function in daily life. If we want to do anything more invigorating then we really need to fuel our muscles. When we eat, we convert carbohydrates (sugars and starches) into glucose (another type of sugar). Glucose stays in the bloodstream and our blood sugar levels rise.

Sensitive beta cells in the pancreas react to this increased glucose and produce a hormone called insulin. Insulin is the catalyst that allows the glucose in our bloodstream to be absorbed into our cells. It is then either converted to energy for immediate use, or stored for the future. As the glucose moves from the bloodstream into the cells, our blood sugar levels drop and the beta cells react accordingly, reducing the creation of insulin.

Normal blood sugar levels therefore fluctuate between 70 and 120 milligrams per decilitre, depending on when it is tested in this cycle; before, during or after eating. High blood sugar levels around 180 straight after a meal, dropping to under 140 within two hours, and falling as low as 70 after several hours of not eating, are considered a normal and healthy range.

2 WHAT IS DIABETES

What is diabetes?

There are two main types of diabetes, but in both forms it this ability to convert food into energy that is compromised.

In Type 1 diabetes, the immune system attacks the cells of the pancreas. Without instruction from the beta cells, the pancreas stops making insulin. This form of the disease usually shows up before the age of 40 and is often triggered by a viral infection.

In Type 2 diabetes, either the pancreas cells do not naturally make enough insulin, or the body's cells cannot use the hormone properly, which is known as insulin resistance. Individuals who develop this type of diabetes often have an underlying genetic susceptibility, but the condition is generally triggered by lifestyle factors such as physical inactivity, obesity and age. Type 2 diabetes tends to present later in life, and in overweight individuals.

The third type is gestational diabetes, which is a form of the disease that only manifests during pregnancy.

In all forms of diabetes, whether the insulin is not

being made or used properly, glucose builds up in the bloodstream after eating instead of being converted into energy. Blood sugar levels in excess of 180 will prompt the kidneys to get rid of the sugar through urination. Common symptoms of diabetes therefore are an unquenchable thirst as a result of excess urination.

The rapid loss of sugar and water leaves a person feeling tired and hungry, and can also result in weight loss. Other warning signs that there is a blood sugar level imbalance include blurred vision, skin infections and wounds that don't heal as a result of poor blood circulation.

Over time, high blood glucose levels can damage many parts of the body, including the heart and blood vessels, eyes, kidneys, nerves, feet, and skin. Complications of diabetes include foot ulcers (see foot care section), skin infections and wounds that won't heal (see skin care section), neuropathy (tingling, numbness or pain due to nerve damage), high blood pressure, liver disease, eye disease or retinopathy, which can lead to blindness. All symptoms should be dealt with as soon as possible to minimise the long-term impact.

3 TRADITIONAL MEDICATIONS

Traditional Medications

Diabetes has been manageable since Eli Lilly and Company manufactured insulin in 1922, but it is considered a chronic condition that is not curable. Type 1 patients typically depend on an injection of external insulin as their bodies no longer produce the hormone. This condition is generally not reversible (although some cases have been claimed), but many sufferers have experienced significant improvements in controlling glucose levels through various alternate methods.

Type 2 patients are typically insulin resistant and many can reverse their diabetes with a significant lifestyle change. Some patients may still require insulin injections if they are unable to control their blood sugar levels, but can still reap the rewards of a new regime of eating and exercising.

Diabetics should aim to keep their blood glucose levels within a healthy range, which can be achieved through a variety of methods including blood glucose monitoring, eating a suitable diet, increasing physical activity and insulin medication. Each sufferer is individual, so what works for one might not be appropriate for another, but there are a number of alternative remedies which some patients have found successful to greater or lesser degrees.

4 FOCUS ON FOOD

Focus on food

Little and often

Getting into the habit of eating little and often will improve your body's ability to regulate sugar levels and won't stress the system by having to process an overload of food at once. Three small meals a day with two light snacks in between, is considered ideal, providing of course that you don't increase your overall calorie intake.

It is also important for diabetics to get to know their own body and how it reacts to different food substances. This can be done using a blood glucose meter to test sugar levels before eating, and at two hourly intervals after a meal. Understanding how the body processes each food type can be a very useful tool to manage your diet and regulate the glucose in your bloodstream.

Low Carb High Fat

The Low Carb High Fat diet originated in Sweden and has a strong following amongst Scandinavians. This diet can be followed for life and has been adopted by diabetics and those simply looking to lose weight alike. The body requires less insulin as the volume of carbohydrates is significantly reduced, but receives vital nutrients through choosing full fat options of allowed food.

The diet is broken down into green, amber and red light foods, which should be eaten freely, consumed in moderation and avoided respectively.

Green light foods should make up the majority of the diet, and cover all dairy, meat, fish and vegetables, with the preference being towards full fat options including leaving fat on meat while cooking. Amber light foods, which can be eaten in moderation, include beans, lentils, nuts, almonds, sunflower seeds, fruit and chocolate with a high cocoa content.

Red light foods are typically high in carbohydrates and sugars and should only be eaten in minimal quantities so as to reduce the need for insulin. This group covers potato, rice, bread, flour and corn based products, cereal-based products such as pasta, pastry, biscuits and breakfast cereals, dried fruit, sweets, cakes, sugary drinks, margarine and omega-6 based oils (corn, sunflower, safflower, soybean and peanut).

Carbohydrate Counting

Cutting carbohydrates out altogether is not advisable as some carbs are important for your overall health. So, rather than just simply avoiding carbs, many diabetics choose a method of counting the carbohydrates they are consuming to understand the effect each food type has on blood sugar levels and the level of medication required as a result.

For diabetics requiring insulin injections, carbohydrate counting is a method of matching the levels of artificial insulin with the carbs in your food and drink. For diabetics who don't need insulin, carb counting can still be useful to monitor the effect of different carbs and affords greater freedom of lifestyle through blood glucose management and a healthy body.

Carbohydrate counting is however a fairly complicated process which requires training from a healthcare professional, scales, patience and diligence. Mastering the technique can not only help a diabetic manage medication, but also understand his or her own body better.

The carbohydrates which tend to have the most pronounced effect on blood sugar levels tend to be starchy carbohydrates such as rice, pasta, bread, potatoes and similar root vegetables, flour based products (pastry, cakes, biscuits, battered food etc) and certain fruits.

Low G.I.

The Glycaemic Index was created to help people understand the relative absorption values of different foods, and diabetics benefit from food which is digested more slowly to manage their blood sugar fluctuations better. Glucose, the body's source of energy, is set at 100 on the GI scale and foods with a lower GI value are therefore preferable to maintain steadier glucose levels.

To some extent, it is possible to swap simple carbs for their more complex counterparts. Complex carbohydrates are considered better dietary choices anyway because of the additional nutrients, and switching white bread, rice and pasta to whole grain versions, eating oat, bran or barley products, and adding vegetables to meals will aid in lowering the glycaemic index of your diet.

However, other factors affect the GI value of food, such as the ripeness, what the food is served with, as well as how it is processed and cooked. So, like counting carbohydrates, this method of monitoring your diet can be complicated and take some time to understand fully. Still, grasping some of the basic concepts is a worthwhile exercise and can help you manage your body's sugar fluctuations.

Tips and tricks include adding vinegar to food to lower the glycaemic response of many substances and, similarly, eating fat with a carbohydrate to slow down digestion (hence the Scandinavian Low Carb High Fat diet). Unrefined complex carbs are also high in fibre, which again reduces the rise of blood glucose. Protein in oily fish and lean meat is also broken down more slowly by the body, leaving you feeling fuller for longer and creating less movement in blood sugar levels.

The downsides of a diet based on a low GI value are the complicated rules that surround each food, the lack of GI information available on packaging and the impracticality of guessing the relative GI value of food in restaurants.

High Fibre

Rather than coping with the complexity of counting carbohydrates or calculating the GI values of each food to eat only those with a low glycaemic index, a high fibre diet helps the body regulate glucose levels simply by eating foods which the body digests more slowly.

Vegetables are a good source of fibre, although it is still best to choose those with low glycaemic index value. The best type of fibre is soluble fibre which can be found in apples, apricots, beets, berries, carrots, citrus fruits, parsnips, and winter squash, among other foods. Oats are also extremely rich in soluble fibre and are a good addition in cereal products and breads.

Soluble fibre has an additional health advantage, which is to lower elevated LDL cholesterol levels. This so called 'bad' cholesterol can often be a problem for diabetics. Nuts are a great source of fibre and vitamins which can help lower cholesterol, but eat them in moderation as they can be calorific.

Any food that is processed from grains, while high in fibre can also have a high concentration of carbohydrate, so it's advisable for diabetics to test their blood sugar level before and after eating a new grain-based product to measure the effect each item has on the body.

Vegan or Vegetarian

There are notably fewer incidences of diabetes among vegetarians or vegans and so studies have been conducted to see if following a meat, fish or dairy-free diet can help the condition. While no conclusions have been drawn just yet, it is known that a healthy balanced diet can significantly improve diabetes.

Both diets can be beneficial for diabetics as saturated fats and cholesterol are cut, while fruit and vegetable intake is increased providing much-needed dietary fibre. However carbohydrates are often the base of many meals in these diets and can cause blood sugar spikes, so monitoring remains an important feature in maintaining healthy glucose levels when following these diets.

Vegan diets are usually based around vegetables, fruit, grains and legumes, but it is important to ensure a balance of protein, carbohydrates, fat, vitamins and minerals is reached, and vitamin B12 supplements are often advisable.

An extreme version of a vegan diet is a completely raw diet, consisting of just vegetables, seeds and nuts. Kirt Tyson famously reversed what was initially thought to be Type 2 diabetes, but in fact turned out to be Type 1, by following a very limited diet of food that is neither cooked nor processed.

As raw recipes tend to be low in fat, consisting mostly of low GI foods that are high in fibre, vitamins and minerals, this type of diet can be beneficial to managing diabetes. However, the diet is also low in some important nutrition elements such as protein, fat, iron, calcium and vitamin D and is not recommended without advice from a healthcare professional to ensure that a healthy nutritional balance is met.

Low Calories

Another extreme form of diet that is gaining popularity among diabetics is the 800 calorie diet which was studied by Newcastle University. Also known as the Newcastle diet, it is often confusingly called the 600 calorie diet due to the way it is administered; 600 calories is provided via a meal replacement sachet, with the remaining 200 calories being consumed through non-starchy vegetables.

Funded by Diabetes UK, the results of the study suggest that the diet makes the body expel fat which has previously been clogging up the pancreas, allowing it the freedom to create insulin again. Many of the participants showed normal blood sugar levels after the 8 week trial and appeared to be cured of Type 2 diabetes, although careful eating and increased exercise were recommended on a daily basis.

A similar, raw vegetable juice-only, diet was tried by Dr Gabriel Cousens' diabetic patients in America to comparable results in less time (one month as opposed to 8 weeks). Very low calorie diets like this should only be undertaken with support from a healthcare professional as side effects can include headaches, dizziness, hunger, tiredness and feeling cold.

5 DIETARY SUPPLEMENTS

Dietary Supplements

Herbs, spices and plant-based supplements

There are a number of natural herbs and spices which can be added into cooking to give flavour, some of which are believed to help control glucose levels. There is limited research on the effectiveness of these substances, but if they are to your taste then it might be interesting to see if they have any stabilising effect on your blood sugar levels.

Aloe Vera

Aloe vera is a product of the succulent plant of the same name and has been used in herbal medicine since the first century. Aloe vera products can be bought in most pharmacies or large supermarkets.

It is widely used in many health and beauty products due to its healing, rejuvenating and soothing properties, and is most commonly used to treat skin complaints. Aloe vera cream can be useful to aid slow-healing wounds which can be a problem for diabetics with poor blood circulation.

The juice is thought to help lower blood lipids, which can be high in Type 2 patients, and improve blood glucose levels. It is also thought to aid the digestive system, specifically treating constipation, and facilitate good dental health. There is no conclusive proof of these claims, with the skin healing qualities being the recognized use of this plant.

Bitter melon

Bitter melon is a vine found across Asia and Africa. The juice, also known as bitter gourd, has been well-connected through research and clinical trials to lower blood sugar levels, although more evidence is needed to be conclusive.

The fruit itself can usually be found in Asian grocery shops and other forms of the supplement can be found in health food stores. It can be eaten as a fruit, made into a juice, the seeds can be ground and added to food, or it can simply be bought as an herbal supplement.

Excessive consumption however can cause mild abdominal pain or diarrhoea, so it is not recommended to add more than two ounces of bitter melon to your diet a day. You should check with your healthcare professional whether or not it is safe to use alongside your current medication, as there is a risk of hypoglycaemia and blood sugar levels should always be monitored while taking this supplement.

Cinnamon

Cinnamon is a sweet, pungent spice derived from the bark of wild cinnamon trees. Found in tropical areas across Southeast Asia, South America and the Caribbean, cinnamon is often used for a warm flavour in cooking and baking in those regions.

Cinnamon has also been the subject of a number of trials and has proven beneficial in lowering glucose levels as well as reducing 'bad' LDL cholesterol and triglycerides. A regular dose of at least half a teaspoon, a few grams, of cinnamon a day is understood to mimic insulin; by softening cell membranes cinnamon increases insulin sensitivity.

Cinnamon is sold in many forms, including cinnamon sticks, powder, tea, oil and tablet supplements (cinnamon extract). Many of these products can be found in larger supermarkets and will be stocked in health stores.

Fenugreek

Fenugreek is an aromatic plant grown in India, North Africa and around the Mediterranean, popular in cooking (predominantly used in curries) and herbal remedies. Initial studies have shown that fenugreek, rich in soluble fibre, can help lower cholesterol and improve glycaemic control, however proven links are absent and most of the good news is anecdotal.

The leaves are either sold fresh, known as methi, or dried as a herb, while the seeds are used both whole and in powdered form as a spice. The leaves and seeds can usually be found in Asian grocery stores, while fenugreek herbal supplements should be available in health stores.

Doses range from 5 grams to 90 grams per day, however there are some concerns that excess consumption (more than 100 grams) can cause an upset stomach, while diarrhoea and wind are common side effects. As with all blood sugar-reducing herbs, it is wise to consult a healthcare professional before embarking on a sustained course of fenugreek.

Ginger

Ginger is a pungent knotted plant stem, native to Africa, India, China, Australia and Jamaica. It is a popular spice added for a warm flavour in Asian cuisine, as well as being used in herbal medicine, typically to aid digestion, combat a cold and relieve pain.

Ginger has been shown to increase the absorption of glucose into cells, as well as improving insulin secretion. A small daily dose has also been seen to slow the progression of cataracts, which is a common sight-related complication of long-term diabetes.

Additionally ginger has a very low glycaemic index which helps regulate glucose levels.

It can be readily bought fresh, dried or powdered in supermarkets, and is available as a supplement or juice in most health stores.

Onion

Onion is a widely available vegetable which is used to add a complementary base flavour to numerous dishes from many cuisines. Onions contain a number of elements which are thought to have anti-inflammatory, anti-cholesterol, anti-cancer and antioxidant properties.

For diabetes, the active compound of allyl propyl disulphide (APDS) in onions is thought to have a dual effect of blocking the breakdown of insulin by the liver, as well as stimulating the pancreas to producing insulin. The result is reduced blood sugar levels, and it is believed to lower 'bad' LDL cholesterol, raise 'good' HDL cholesterol, and help prevent heart disease.

Fresh onions can easily be found in any general store, market or supermarket and can be used fresh or cooked in all manner of recipes. Cutting onions releases a number of acids which can irritate the eye and be temporarily uncomfortable, so you can even buy frozen, pre-chopped onions. There are a number of varieties, such as red onion or shallots, and you can also buy onion powder if you like the taste, but not the texture.

6 MINERAL AND VITAMIN SUPPLEMENTS

Mineral and vitamin supplements

Mineral or vitamin supplements are usually available in tablet, capsule, powder and liquid forms. They are intended to provide additional nutrients missing in a healthy diet, and should not be consumed instead of fresh food or in large quantities to correct an on-going deficiency.

ALA and GLA

Alpha-lipoic acid (ALA) is a powerful natural antioxidant found in foods such as liver, spinach, broccoli and potatoes. Inconclusive studies have been conducted to understand its effect on insulin and glucose, but it is known to treat diabetic neuropathy as it helps protect against cell damage.

Gamma-lipoic acid (GLA) is another natural antioxidant, found in evening primrose oil, borage oil and blackcurrant seed oil. It is also used to treat nerve damage caused by diabetic neuropathy. These supplements are available as tablets or capsules from most health stores.

Chromium

Chromium is a mineral which is essential to the human body in small quantities. It is found in a number of foods including brewer's yeast, meat, chicken, shellfish (especially clams), corn oil and whole grain products. Some studies have shown links between increased chromium and improved glucose tolerance, particularly when combined with niacin. However it is likely to be most effective for people with a natural deficiency in the mineral, or depleted levels caused by age, strenuous exercise or physiological trauma.

Chromium is available in capsule and tablet supplements as chromium picolinate, chromium chloride and chromium nicotinate, but there is not enough proof yet of its benefits to recommend it for diabetes management. As with other blood sugar-reducing supplements caution should be taken in using chromium as high doses can cause serious side effects, including kidney problems. High levels of niacin might also block glucose tolerance, so medical advice should be sought and blood sugar levels monitored while taking the supplement.

Magnesium

There is a strong indication of a link between magnesium deficiency and insulin resistance, but numerous trials of increased magnesium in diabetic patients have produced mixed results and inconsistent reactions over several decades.

Despite the lack of clarity and understanding, many doctors would still advise a magnesium-rich diet for diabetics, but it is best to discuss this with your healthcare professional before taking such a step and to keep a close watch on your blood sugar levels.

Vitamin B

The vitamin B group plays an important role in cell metabolism; B1 is key to releasing energy from carbohydrates, B3 has two structures which are both needed to transfer energy from glucose, fat and alcohol consumption, and B6, B7 and B12 are all involved in metabolism of carbohydrates, lipids, amino acids and proteins.

Some studies suggest that vitamin B6 may be able to improve glucose tolerance, particularly in gestational diabetes and where intolerance is caused by birth control pills.

However there are also strong links between vitamin B and the treatment of diabetic neuropathy. Vitamin B12 in particular, along with vitamins B1 and B6, is critical for nerve cells to function normally. Supplements of these vitamins for people suffering with damaged nerve endings have proven very successful in reducing and managing the associated pain.

Vitamin C

Vitamin C is an essential nutrient which acts as a catalyst for a number of different enzyme reactions. It is a weak sugar acid with a similar structure to glucose, a deficiency in which would usually present as scurvy. The group of vitamins plays different roles in the two main types of diabetes.

Type 1 sufferers with low vitamin C levels may have increased amounts of sorbitol in their system, which is a harmful sugar that leads to common diabetic complications such as retinopathy, neuropathy and kidney damage.

Type 2 diabetics who increase their vitamin C consumption can improve glucose tolerance and reduce urinary protein loss, as well as lowering sorbitol levels.

Vitamin D

Vitamin D is produced naturally in the body in response to the sun's rays and can be found in a variety of foods such as nuts, oily fish, eggs, powdered milk and some fortified cereals. It plays a number of important roles in the body from maintaining the health of bones, teeth and joints, to assisting the immune system. It is also thought that raising vitamin D in the body can help to keep blood glucose levels under control.

Additional benefits of vitamin D which can help diabetics are to regulate the appetite, lower hunger levels and avoid sweet snacks. It can also reduce levels of cortisol; this stress hormone can lead to increased abdominal fat when high quantities are maintained over a sustained period, which is a key factor in developing Type 2 diabetes. Vitamin D3 is far more effective than vitamin D2, but most supplements available in pharmacies, health stores and supermarkets contain the hugely inferior vitamin D2, so it is always worth checking the label.

Zinc

Chemically similar to magnesium, zinc is an essential mineral and a zinc deficiency is thought to be associated with many diseases. One such believed outcome is to contribute to the development of diabetes, as it is thought to be a crucial element in insulin metabolism.

Zinc is well-known to support the immune system and ward off viral infections, but it may also offer protection to beta cells from internal destruction. Although there are no proven beneficial links, doctors often recommend a zinc supplement to diabetics.

7 HERBAL REMEDIES

Herbal remedies

The health market is flooded with herbal remedies, all claiming to beneficial for one thing or another and in fact many claim to be a 'cure all' for almost anything. Some of the more creditable claims are noted here, but it is important to continue with other medication and traditional treatment while trying some of these supplements and monitor your blood sugar levels carefully in case they cause a reaction. Equally, if you are keeping a close eye on your glucose, you may see an improvement or stabilisation when you introduce one of the substances, in which case you may choose to continue with the herbal remedy.

Blueberry Leaves

Blueberry leaves are a common remedy for age-related diabetes. The active compound, Myrillin, helps to increase capillary strength, which is something that typically depletes with age. This in turn improves the vascular system and reduces the free-radical change in cells.

Curry Leaves

Curry leaves, from the tree of the same name in India, are another herb used in traditional Ayurvedic medicine for diabetes. They are believed to help regulate sugar levels in the blood and urine, but as curry leaves can also be effective in weight management they are often prescribed to prevent obesity and therefore the related Type 2 diabetes.

Coccinia indica

Also known as "ivy gourd", coccinia indica has traditionally been used in Ayurverdic remedies. Further studies are needed, but initial results suggest that the herb mimics the function of insulin and can therefore have a positive effect on glycaemic control.

Fig Leaves

Fig leaves are used in a number of homemade remedies and are particularly popular in Spain and south west Europe as a treatment for diabetes. A few studies on animals suggest that fig leaves might aid glucose uptake, but there is no conclusive evidence to support this claim. Common ways to take the herb are a portion of fig leaf extract with breakfast or boiling the leaves in water and drinking it like a tea.

Glucomannan

Glucomannan is a dietary fibre supplement that can be used by diabetics as it delays the process of the stomach emptying, which in turn moderates the rate of glucose uptake. Some studies have shown that blood sugar levels straight after a meal are lower in diabetics who have been given glucomannan in their food. It is also suggested that glucomannan may be particularly beneficial in pregnancy-related diabetes. Glucomannan is available in capsules and should be taken before eating.

Grape seed Extract

Grape seed extract is a supplement which has been shown in a few studies to protect the liver cells and to create a defence mechanism against hyperglycaemic conditions. The extract can be bought in capsules for ease and it is suggested that you take 50mg per 50 lbs of weight, not exceeding 300mg per day.

Gymnema

Gymnema is a woody shrub whose leaves suppress a sweet tooth and are believed to help lower blood sugar level. A number of animal studies have led to a variety of theories on what the active ingredient is and, while there is no conclusion as to how, it is generally believed to raise insulin levels.

Hibiscus

Hibiscus is a large flowering plant in the mallow family and features in traditional Indian treatments for diabetes. There are a few preliminary studies which support hibiscus being beneficial to diabetics. Dried flowers are added to boiling water and made into a tea, to be taken three times a day.

Mango Leaves

Mango is a popular fruit from South Asia, but the leaves are shown to lower blood sugar levels. Fresh leaves can be soaked overnight in water, or dried leaves can be mixed with water, to be taken as a solution both morning and night.

8 LET'S GET PHYSICAL

Let's get physical

Increased activity

Being overweight is one of the typical causes of Type 2 diabetes and therefore any increase in physical activity is recommended to help lose weight and regain a healthy body. In addition to losing weight, regular exercise and enhanced muscle movement can help achieve greater control of blood sugar levels as cells increase their sugar uptake for fuel.

There are many further benefits of regular exercise as it tones up all muscles, including the heart which can help reduce the risk of heart disease. Lung capacity also improves, HDL 'good' cholesterol levels are raised and LDL 'bad' cholesterol levels are lowered, while bones and joints are strengthened. Emotional benefits are seen alongside the physical improvements and blood pressure can be lowered as levels of stress and tension are decreased.

A healthy amount of exercise is usually defined as either two and a half hours of moderate intensity physical activity, or one and a quarter hours of high intensity exercise per week. Moderate intensity means an increased heart rate and sweating, while high intensity would be out of breath and unable to hold a conversation while exercising. However, if you are overweight it is always better to build up slowly by doing a little moderate exercise more frequently.

If you are new to exercise or conscious of your size, you don't have to parade yourself in Lycra down at your local gym, you could try any of the following instead: brisk walking, cycling on flat roads, jogging, swimming, hiking or rambling. Once you improve your fitness, you might like to try increasing the intensity and step up to hill cycling, running, swimming continuous lengths, or climbing.

If you don't have the willpower to do it on your own, you could coerce a friend to join you, or your local gym will usually offer a personal trainer who can induct and motivate you on a range of cardio and weight machines. There are also any number of classes you could join, try the full range from aerobics and dance, to toning and self-defence to see what suits you best.

Precautions

While healthcare professionals would almost always recommend exercise, diabetics do need to be aware of a few precautions and would be wise to consult with a doctor first to design a suitable programme.

As exercise uses glucose to create energy, it is crucial to learn how to balance food, exercise and medication to prevent your blood glucose levels from dropping too low. It is also important to stay hydrated and ensure you eat carbohydrates before exercise and have a fast-acting carbohydrate available, such as glucose tablets, during any activity, to prevent hypoglycaemia.

Additionally if you suffer from poor circulation, as is common in diabetics, it may be wise to avoid high-impact activities which could have the potential for a foot injury (see foot care section). Intense exercise can also threaten eyes already weakened by diabetes, so should be avoided for people susceptible to such issues. Increased exercise usually leads to additional showers, so it is important not to let the skin become dry (see skin care section).

It is advisable to wear a form of diabetic identification if you are exercising alone, or making someone in your class or gym aware of your condition, so that you can get the best help in case of an emergency.

Weightlifting

Aerobic exercise is the traditionally recommended activity to combat diabetes, but recent studies on male exercise patterns have demonstrated the benefits of weightlifting. Many people can find cardio exercise difficult for a number of reasons, and so weight lifting may be more accessible, particularly to those who are overweight.

While aerobic exercise is considered synonymous with weight loss, weightlifting has other benefits. By exhausting a specific group of muscles at once, it encourages cells to increase sugar take-up while also reducing the levels of plasma-free fatty acids. High-impact aerobics, such as running, is notoriously bad for joints in the long term, whereas weightlifting actively strengthens the muscles, which in turn helps to protect bones and joints from injury.

In order to ensure that you are holding yourself in the right position, and therefore targeting the right muscles, you should start by getting some advice from a local gym or personal trainer. Begin by lifting a weight you can manage without too much strain, and repeat each exercise up to 15 times. You can then gradually build up the weight when you can do more than 15 repetitions easily, but you must always make sure that you are in control and not snatching at the weight. Work different muscle groups throughout the week allowing recovery and repair time.

Yoga

Yoga is another excellent alternative to aerobic exercise as it gently stretches and tones the body, improves circulation, relaxes the mind and massages the internal organs. It is accessible to everyone, even those with disabilities, and can be enjoyed free at home or in the social environment of a class.

Start with some breathing exercises to put you in the right frame of mind, as yoga is as much a mental workout as a physical one. Once you are ready there are a number of poses which are believed to be particularly suitable for diabetics as they are supposed to aid digestion, activate kidney functions and increase metabolism.

Downward Facing Dog is a well-known and fairly basic pose which helps with flexibility and toning the muscles, as well as calming the body and mind, which in turn alleviates high blood pressure. The forward bend also aids digestion and encourages blood circulation to the liver and kidneys, which are vulnerable in diabetics. As well as other standing bends such as Triangle, there are a number of sitting bends which offer similar benefits, but might prove easier for beginners.

There are numerous twisting poses which are said to stimulate internal organs, aid digestion and promote blood circulation. Try the Half Lord of Fishes, Dragonfly, Locust and Fish poses, or any of the Marichi series. While some of these exercises look complex, there are always options for beginners and you will be surprised how quickly you will improve with regular practice.

Finally, the Western Intense pose is traditionally believed to reduce obesity and strengthen pelvic floor muscles, which can be weakened in diabetic women.

Twisting poses are not recommended for people with high blood pressure and some poses that cross the legs also might not be suitable if you suffer from poor circulation to the feet. With this in mind it is advisable to get some personalised advice to create a yoga programme that suits you.

9 SKIN CARE

Skin care

The excessive levels of sugar in the diabetic's bloodstream provide a breeding ground for bacteria and fungi, which can lead to skin problems and reduce the body's ability to heal.

There are a couple of reasons why a diabetic's skin can be dry. Sustained high blood sugar levels prompt the kidneys to remove glucose through excess urination. This loss of fluid dehydrates the body and leaves the skin dry while other, more essential, organs take the remaining water. Equally, diabetic neuropathy can damage the nerve endings, particularly in the legs. These faulty nerve endings can prevent messages getting around the body to produce sweat. Without the natural moisturiser of sweating, skin can become dry.

Dry skin is prone to becoming red, sore and itchy. Subconscious scratching to relieve the irritant can result in cracks appearing in the skin, which then allows infection to enter the body. As diabetes can prevent self-healing, once the skin is broken it can take a lot longer than normal to heal. If not treated properly, this can lead to severe complications.

A few simple precautionary steps can be taken to look after the skin and prevent any such problems. Bathe or shower in warm, not hot, water and use a moisturised soap or shower gel. Don't spend too long in the water and pat yourself dry, rather than rubbing. Ensure you dry yourself fully, and then follow up with a light, unscented moisturiser all over. Keep a moisturiser by your sink so that you can reapply to your hands each time after washing. If your skin does become dry, use a moisturiser to relieve the itching, rather than scratching.

Always protect the skin from the sun, using a minimum of SPF 15 cream all year round, and cover exposed areas such as face and ears in the cold wind. Lip balm can help prevent chapped lips in the heat or cold wind. If you notice any persistent problems, see your healthcare provider as soon as possible to get treatment early.

10 FOOT CARE

Foot care

It is important to take the above precautions for skin care in general, but it is even more critical for diabetics to take extra special care of the feet. Damaged nerves can mean a cut on the foot goes unnoticed, while poor circulation and excess blood sugar can impede the healing process.

Unchecked, a simple cut on a foot can lead to serious complications. You should inspect your feet daily or at least weekly, have an annual check-up with a healthcare provider and seek medical attention early if you do get a foot ulcer, cut or other injury.

Ensure that you wash your feet daily and dry thoroughly, but gently, between each toe. Keep toenails trimmed and filed so that they do not cut other toes or become ingrown. Regular foot checks can alert you to any red spots, cuts, swelling or blisters. See a podiatrist to deal with any corns, calluses, verrucas or other foot problems, rather than trying to treat them yourself.

Apply a thin layer of moisturiser to the soles of your feet daily, not between the toes, and always wear comfortable shoes and socks to prevent cuts. Always protect your feet from extreme heat (such as sand on the beach, or a hot bath) and cold (keep warm in the winter).

Keep the blood flowing to your feet, by being active, raising your feet when sitting, wriggling your toes and rotating your ankles a few times a day and avoiding crossing your legs.

11 PHYSICAL TREATMENTS

Physical treatments

Acupuncture

What is it?

Acupuncture is a traditional Chinese medical practice that dates back thousands of years. It is believed that the body's natural energy flow can get blocked, and trained practitioners can release this qi (pronounced "chee") through inserting small, thin needles into various pulse points on the body. There are over 400 specific acupuncture sites from head to toe, and the area treated is not always the same as the area affected.

How can it help?

Some scientists believe that acupuncture induces the body to produce natural painkillers. There is some evidence to support this idea and the method has been shown to offer relief from chronic pain. Therefore, it can often be recommended for use by diabetics suffering from with neuropathy.

Additionally the acupuncture points for the pancreas

can be stimulated to improve functionality. Moderate diabetes often responds to a combination of diet, exercise and acupuncture.

What are the risks?

The risks of acupuncture are limited, but it is essential to visit a trained and registered practitioner as the practice pierces the skin. Diabetics undergoing acupuncture should take extra care of the skin treated and it is recommended to balance this traditional alternate practice with modern Western medication.

Acupressure

What is it?

Acupressure uses the same principle of acupoints as acupuncture to release the body's natural flow of energy. Instead of small needles, physical pressure is applied to the relevant points with a hand, elbow or other blunt instrument.

How can it help?

This traditional Chinese method is less common and so the benefits are not as well documented. It is believed that there are a few relief points for diabetics along the top of the spine, but a fuller study has yet to be completed.

What are the risks?

As acupressure does not pierce the skin there are fewer risks, but extra skin care on the treated areas is still recommended and this practice should also be undertaken in combination with modern medication.

Massage

What is it?

Massage used to be the ultimate luxury pampering treat, reserved only for special occasions. However the health benefits of regular massage have been well-documented and it can even help diabetes' sufferers. Masseurs manipulate and knead muscles to ease pain and tension, while relaxing the body and mind in a soothing environment.

How can it help?

Massage therapy can provide physical as well as mental well-being for diabetics, as it helps to lower both stress levels and blood pressure. Massage can also have direct results by improving blood circulation and relieving symptoms of diabetic neuropathy. It is also thought to stimulate the brain's vagus nerve, causing the secretion of food-absorption hormones, including insulin.

What are the risks?

With very few medical risks associated to massage, it is an additional health care option that is easy to access, and can be shared with a partner or friend as part of a spa day treat.

Reflexology

What is it?

Reflexology is a specialist massage which is usually performed on the feet. The practice focuses on the manipulation of a wide variety of isolated reflex points on the feet which relate to different parts of the body. Through matching a number of techniques with the various reflex points, the practitioner aims to balance the whole body, as well as relieving specific points of discomfort, tension or damage.

How can it help?

As well as promoting a general feeling of health and vitality, reflexology can focus on localised symptoms of poor circulation and neuropathy. A treatment programme might work on improving the wellness of the pancreas and hormone system as a whole, with the aim to encourage natural production of insulin.

Similarly the liver could be targeted to improve its function to counteract the increased blood sugar levels. Finally it could be used to treat specific symptoms which could include the digestive system, to reduce nausea, or the urinary system, to help with the excessive urination.

What are the risks?

Neuropathy, or diabetic nerve damage, leaves feet vulnerable to unknown damage as blisters, corns, calluses and injuries might not be felt. It is important to check the condition of your feet regularly and although reflexology can help circulation it is not advisable to get treatment until any wounds are healed.

Spinal Manipulation

What is it?

Chiropractors practice spinal manipulation in order to align bones, joints, muscles and the spine. These adjustments optimise neural connections throughout the body to improve health and relieve pain. Spinal manipulation is traditionally used to treat back and neck pain, and despite claims to cure other ailments nothing further has yet been proven.

How can it help?

Misalignments in the spine, known as vertebral subluxations, can prevent the nerve supply running efficiently from the upper neck or middle back down to the pancreas. It is believed that if the pancreatic function is disturbed in this way, it may affect its ability to produce enzymes to digest proteins, fats and carbohydrates, or even insulin. Therefore chiropractic adjustments focus on reducing these subluxations, which improves the co-ordination of the nervous system and organs.

What are the risks?

There are few risks related to spinal manipulation, but it should be considered as part of an overall treatment plan which would include a change of diet and increased exercise, as well as medication if required.

In some instances it can pose a risk for patients of stroke or artery and nerve-related damage, so caution should be taken for diabetic patients suffering with neuropathy.

Relaxation practices

Alternative health solutions are becoming increasingly common for a number of reasons. Scepticism is giving way to case studies as practitioners are undertaking and documenting trials to prove correlation. Drugs can be expensive if not funded, particularly if required several times daily, and many people do not like taking being dependant on daily injections or pills. While there is no proven method to cure diabetes, different methods work for difference people. No matter how bizarre some of the practices may sound, don't dismiss them without further investigation as it might just be the one that helps you.

Aromatherapy

What is it?

Aromatherapy is an ancient alternative treatment based on the use of essential oils to improve the patient's health and mood. Each oil has its own effect on the body which include stimulating, relaxing, sedating, decongesting and inflammation reduction. Oils are administered through massage, a vaporiser, on a tissue under the nose or in a bath.

How can it help?

Essential oils cannot help with the control of blood

sugar levels, however aromatherapy massage can significantly aid poor circulation which is often a problem associated with diabetes. There is also suggestion that a combination of oils can help reduce infections which take longer to heal in diabetics.

What are the risks?

The side effects are minimal, but it is advisable to consult your diabetes healthcare provider before undertaking any treatment to ensure there is no clash with your current medication.

Biofeedback

What is it?

Biofeedback is an alternative therapy that promotes stress reduction and relaxation techniques. The practice is based on mind-over-matter, and the principle that we can improve the health of our body through mind power and increased body awareness. Machines record muscle contractions and skin temperatures to help the patient understand his or her own body's reactions, with the ultimate aim being to learn to control them.

How can it help?

Lowering levels of stress is beneficial to diabetes by reducing the blood sugar levels, as well as the other emotional and physical benefits reaped from learning to relax. Biofeedback helps a patient become more aware of their body, its reactions and how to manage pain, which can also help with diabetic neuropathy.

What are the risks?

As a new therapy it has not been validated as an effective technique, but it can be useful for stress management and body awareness without any side effects.

Colour, Music and Art Therapy

What is it?

Colour, music and art therapies are all new experimental techniques using creativity to communicate with the patient and promote relaxation.

How can it help?

These therapies are commonly used for patients with mental health issues or learning difficulties, but they are also used in palliative care and may be able to help with pain relief and complications arising from diabetes.

What are the risks?

There are no known risks and, although the validity has not yet been established, devoted practitioners say they have happy patients who benefit from this discipline.

Guided Imagery

What is it?

Guided imagery is a new practice which helps stroke victims regain lost abilities through visualisation to improve the connection between the mind and body. By focussing the mind on the activity, there is evidence that this promotes the brain to physically perform the activity. It can also be used as a relaxation technique, using peaceful imagery to calm the body physically.

How can it help?

Relaxation therapy such as guided imagery can be useful for people who suffer with chronic conditions to manage stress and relax both the body and mind. It is believed that patients with an optimistic outlook will have better health. Visualisation helps create a positive mental image which helps the patient manage, and improve, their own perception of diabetes.

What are the risks?

There are no risks to this form of relaxation therapy and it can be performed by anyone, anywhere, so it is a good technique for sufferers of chronic conditions, such as diabetes, to maintain a healthy outlook on life.

Homeopathy

What is it?

Homeopathy practitioners follow the principle that "like cures like", i.e. a substance which is bad in large quantities, can be beneficial in small doses. Each patient is individually analysed and prescribed a combination of substances designed to realign and balance the body to cure symptoms of diseases.

How can it help?

Insulin might be prescribed orally as 10 or 20 drops daily administered in water. Other substances such as curare, codenium and syzygium might be tried, along with phosphorous, all with the aim of lowering blood sugar levels.

What are the risks?

The fact that the quantities used are so small and treatments are so individual, makes it very difficult to evaluate the effectiveness of homeopathy. As homeopathic remedies shouldn't have any side effects, it is often considered harmless to try a personalised plan, but it is always safer to try it under the instruction of a healthcare professional rather than self-medicating.

Hypnotherapy

What is it?

A patient is relaxed into a hypnotic state, at which point it is possible for the hypnotist to make an unconscious change in the patient's mind, so that he or she forms new responses, thoughts, attitudes or behaviours to a situation. This technique is commonly used to improve the health and well-being of a patient, specifically to help someone stop smoking, lose weight or overcome fears. It is also gaining a reputation for successful stress relief and pain management.

How can it help?

Hypnotherapy would commonly be used to help diabetic patients lose much-needed weight and start exercising, to ease their condition. It can also help change an attitude towards the illness if depression over having a chronic condition is a problem. More recent studies suggest that hypnosis might also help create a biological reaction within the body which stimulates the nervous system. Such claims are not supported medically, but some patients suggest that they have benefitted from this technique.

What are the risks?

Studies show that while hypnosis doesn't work for everyone, a patient with an open mind should experience some degree of success. There are no real side effects, other than financial, if you don't feel it works. Some patients can feel vulnerable, but a registered practitioner should alleviate any fears.

Meditation

What is it?

Meditation is a mental and breathing technique to manage stress and restore calm; the patient focuses on slow, regular breaths while clearing the mind of distractions. It can be performed anywhere, either by the patient alone, with a tutor or while listening to a recorded track.

How can it help?

Stress is a risk factor in developing Type 2 diabetes among other long-term diseases. The body's natural functions change when put under stress as it prepares itself for "fight or flight". Hormones such as adrenaline are pumped into your body, your heart rate increases and your blood vessels dilate. Your metabolism is slowed down to provide additional glucose in the blood system, ready to be converted into fuel should it be needed. Continued stress can elevate blood sugar levels more often, making control or regulation difficult. Any technique which helps to reduce stress levels will help manage blood sugar levels. Meditation not only helps the mental control of stress, but also slows the breathing which helps to slow the body down physically.

What are the risks?

Meditation is so widely practised because of the far-reaching benefits without drawbacks. By reducing stress levels, meditation can help relieve depression, insomnia and anxiety, as well as lowering the risk for diseases such as heart disease, stroke and hypertension.

12 HOLISTIC APPROACHES

Holistic approaches

Ayurveda

What is it?

Ayurveda is an ancient Indian holistic practice which combines the use of herbs, diet, breathing, massage and meditation to restore balance to the whole body. As well as treatment of illness, the philosophy focuses on maintaining a healthy prana, or life energy, through regular practice. An individual plan is completed for each patient, recommending a unique combination of multidiscipline treatments.

How can it help?

Ayurvedic treatment for diabetes will be individual, but would commonly start with a modified diet eliminating sugar and favouring complex over simple carbohydrates. A cleansing programme called Panchkarma would typically recommend a combination of massage, herbal therapy, saunas and fasting, followed by yoga and breathing exercises. Bitter gourd and fenugreek are two of the common ingredients found in Ayurvedic remedies for diabetes.

What are the risks?

Many of the Ayurveda relaxation practices are safe, sensible measures to maintain a healthy body and mind. There is no scientific evidence to support the herbal remedies and some of the natural supplements have heavy metal content, which can interfere with other medication. Therefore, it is always recommended to seek the consent of a medical professional before undertaking a personalised Ayurvedic plan.

Traditional Chinese Medicine (TCM)

What is it?

Traditional Chinese Medicine (TCM) is an ancient form of holistic treatment comprising a variety of methods including acupuncture, moxibustion, herbal medicine, diet therapy, mind and body exercises, and massage. The human body and mind are viewed as a whole and no part is considered in isolation. TCM is gradually gaining acceptance in the western world, but is usually considered in addition to, rather than instead of, modern medicine.

How can it help?

TCM treatments for diabetes concentrate on improving blood circulation and relieving pain from diabetic neuropathy, although some practices can be of help to stabilise blood sugar levels. Acupuncture or acupressure is typically used to stimulate the pancreas and nervous system. Herbal remedies such as ginseng, balsam pear and guava leaves are given to lower blood glucose levels and raise the spirits. Dietary advice is given to increase intake of "cooling agents" such as vegetables and grains, and reduce sweet substances. Smaller, more frequent meals are recommended at regular times each day. Mind and body balance is achieved through a number of meditational exercises.

What are the risks?

Many relaxation elements of TCM are safe for most patients, but acupuncture is a practice that should be used with caution by diabetics with poor circulation. Acupressure can be used instead which applies physical pressure, rather than needles, to the relevant acupoints. It is advisable to continue with medication and blood sugar monitoring alongside TCM and inform your healthcare professional that you are trying alternative medicine, as some drug-herb interactions can have side effects, particularly in women with gestational diabetes.

www.ingramcontent.com/pod-product-compliance
Lightning Source LLC
Chambersburg PA
CBHW070327290526
45791CB00003B/1290